DON'T TOUCH THE BABY:

A Guide to Touching Babies That Don't Belong to You

Danielle Botz

DEDICATION

This book is dedicated to my people. Thanks for laughing at my jokes, and encouraging me to follow my dreams. I love you all so much.

CONTENTS

CHAPTER ONE:
INTRODUCTORY QUESTIONS

When it comes to touching, kissing, or otherwise handling babies, there are two questions that are vital to ask. Ask yourself these two questions prior to ANY PHYSICAL INTERACTION with a baby.

1. *Is this my baby?*

2. *Do I have permission from the baby's parent or guardian to touch this baby?*

If you cannot answer yes to one of these questions, please take the following actions.

1. **Do not** touch the baby.
2. *Do not* touch the baby.

Included in the back of this booklet is a section for notes. Feel free to use those pages to write out or brainstorm any of the more complicated elements that we will cover in this and future chapters.

CHAPTER TWO:
SPECIAL EXCEPTIONS

Sometimes, a baby does not technically belong to you, but could still be a baby you are allowed to touch. If you THINK this may be the case, consult the following list of questions.

1. *Are you related to this baby?*
2. *Do you know this baby?*
3. *Do you know this baby's parents?*
4. *Did someone who is responsible for the baby ASK you to touch him or her?*
5. *Did you bring this baby to his or her*

current location?

If you cannot answer "yes" to any of these questions, special exception does not apply to you. Please refer to the recommended actions in Chapter One.

CHAPTER 3: WHEN TO PLACE YOUR FILTHY HANDS ON OR AROUND A BABY'S MOUTH

NEVER.

Again, this rule applies to all persons not owning, knowing, or otherwise belonging to the baby in question. If you feel you have reached that message in error, ask yourself the following questions:

1. *Am I a doctor?*
2. *Am I a dentist?*
3. *Am I a medical or dental professional of any kind?*
4. *Am I actively involved in saving this baby's life?*

If you cannot answer "Yes" to any of the above questions, you do not meet the criteria for touching a baby's mouth. Take your hands away. No, you don't need to check to see if they have a tooth coming in, and it is not necessary to place a finger in a baby's mouth to see if they are hungry.

CHAPTER FOUR:
CAN I KISS THE BABY?

No.

Here is a brief, but compelling list of reasons why kissing babies that do not belong to you is a bad idea:

1. Respiratory Syncytial Virus (RSV)- According to the CDC, for children under the age of 5, there are more than 57,000 hospitalizations, 500,000 ER visits, and 1.5 million visits to outpatient clinics each year in the United States.[1] While death from RSV is less common, the infection is

painful, traumatic, and dangerous for babies and their parents/ guardians. Just because something probably won't kill you, doesn't mean it's OK for a stranger to give it to you. Getting punched in the face also won't kill you, but as a society, we've come to frown upon it. Usually.

2. HSV-1 (Also Known as the Cold Sore Virus)- Even if you don't actively have a cold sore, you can spread this virus onto a newborn. If contracted, HSV-1 can quickly cause illness in newborns. It can cause lethargy, seizures, and can even result in the baby's death.[2]

3. Measles- In 2019, Measles cases were confirmed in 31 states, according to CDC.[3] A child following the typical recommended vaccine schedule, will not receive their first dose of the MMR vaccine until 12 months old. And despite the fact that many believe Measles to be "just a rash", there are a host of more serious complications, which include

pneumonia and encephalitis, both of which can lead to death. Children under the age of 5, and adults over the age of 20 are more likely to experience serious complications from contracting the disease.[4] Though death is not necessarily a common side effect of these diseases, for the parents of the baby you just want to snuggle/kiss/hug/touch sooo badly, it's likely not worth the risk. In the case of the diseases listed, as well as many other illnesses, you don't have to be symptomatic in order to pass germs onto another person. That adorable baby you just have touch? He or she won't be so adorable when they're up all night with a fever, or broken out in hives, or hooked up to a ventilator at the hospital. Don't. Touch. Other. People's. Babies.

1. https://wwwn.cdc.gov/nndss/conditions/respiratory-syncytial-virusassociated-mortality/case-definition/2019/
2. .https://www.health.ny.gov/diseases/communicable/herpes/newborns/fact_sheet.htm

3. https://www.cdc.gov/measles/cases-outbreaks.html
4. https://www.cdc.gov/vaccines/vpd/mmr/public/index.html

CHAPTER FIVE:
CONCLUSION

I know that we have covered a lot of very complex topics in this booklet. Because of that, I would like to take this opportunity to summarize the key points concerning the touching of babies that you may encounter out in the world.

1. Do not touch babies that you encounter out in the world unless special circumstances apply.
2. In most cases, special circumstances do not apply.

CHAPTER SIX:
FAQ

Frequently Asked Questions Regarding the Touching of Babies That do not Belong to You:

1. What if the baby is sooo cute?:

This is a great question. If you find yourself in this situation, make sure you do not touch the baby.

2. What if I just touch the baby's hand?:

Another GREAT question. In this case, you are going to want to ask yourself a couple of questions. If you answer "No" to even one of them, please see the answer to question 1 above.

> 1. *Could this hand somehow end up in the baby's mouth?*
> 2. *Is this baby mine?*

3. What if I really really want to snuggle this baby?:

Don't.

A NOTE FROM THE AUTHOR

About 6 months ago, I brought my 8-month-old daughter to the grocery store with me. She was sleeping peacefully in her car seat when a woman I do not know approached my daughter, and without permission, request, or provocation of any kind, placed her hands on my daughter's mouth. This was done in an attempt to either see her tiny lips, or check to see if my daughter had teeth. To be honest, I blacked out for a second and am not sure. I quickly removed the woman's hand and rushed away, but the encounter left me frustrated.

I was a single foot away, picking out some sandwich meat when a person came up to my sleeping baby and put hands of indeterminate cleanliness in and around her mouth. From this experience, this rant was born.

This booklet applies to babies that do not belong to you. It is not intended for parents, guardians, grandparents, or other caregivers or medical professionals. This book is a guide for strangers encountering babies and other small children out in public.

To be honest, I love that so many people want to show love to the babies. The world needs love—now more than ever—but there are lots of ways to interact with strangers that don't include potentially making them sick.

Notes:

DON'T TOUCH THE BABY

DON'T TOUCH THE BABY

DON'T TOUCH THE BABY

DON'T TOUCH THE BABY

DON'T TOUCH THE BABY

www.ingramcontent.com/pod-product-compliance
Lightning Source LLC
Chambersburg PA
CBHW031510210526
45463CB00008B/3176